No more

Jet Lag

Or the Fun of Subsonic Air Travel

Chris Soebroto
Visit us at:
www.nomore-jetlag.com

Cover design by the author

First edition: Jetlag, 2004, Galang Press, Indonesia
Second and expanded edition: 2006

Dedicated to Jonathan Livingston Seagull for successfully overcoming physical limitations associated with flight.

Contents

Chapter	Page

Preface

This book is about jet lag and (air) travel induced anxiety. Jet lag is not a minor discomfort. It's a health issue. That's why this book demystifies modern air travel, especially in Economy or Coach Class.

Fortunately, preventing jet lag is easy. No need to buy fancy gadgets or drugs. All you need to beat jet lag are:

· Your watch
· Eyeshades
· Earplugs
· An inflatable pillow
· A laid back attitude when flying
· This book

Have fun reading and have a safe trip next time. Without jet lag, of course.

Chris Soebroto

A Window Seat

T he very first flight I ever made was a so-called 'camping flight' to Barcelona, Spain. It was a two hours trip in a very noisy propeller driven DC-6. It was a cheap charter flight for backpackers who brought along their camping gear. There is hardly a memory of the outbound leg to Barcelona. It's probably because we had a few beers on the way to the airport in order to generate the right vacation spirit. That worked very well. Later there was a lot more beer in Lloret de Mar, I remember.

At the end of the holiday there was Alicia, a beautiful Spanish girl who studied in France and whose French was impeccable with a very sweet Spanish accent. After one hour of chatting with Alicia my French was amazingly fluent too. Ah, how sweet it was to fall in love in the last few hours of the camping trip before going home. Pending the conversation I reduced the beer ratio significantly. That explains why on the return flight I was very sober. I also had a window seat. Flying across France in the middle of the night at low altitude (12,000 feet or so) I watched the lights of towns and villages as they slowly passed underneath the plane. I could see the headlights of cars winding their way through France. Everything down below was so tiny and looked so peaceful. People there were minding their own business going to the night shift or coming home late from a party. Truck drivers rushed along freeways. It was like floating through heaven on metal wings. From my elevation it was hard to imagine that individuals down below, in the real world, were cheating and scheming and making love. It was hard to imagine that secret deals were being made some-where and that there was war in several places on the globe. As a result of these thoughts, although it was in the middle of summer I quickly came in something of a Christmas mood, wishing peace and good will for all mankind.

That slow flight made me want for more and two years later I found myself checking in for my first long haul flight. It was to become one of the longest long haul flights in my life. I had just graduated and decided to see the world, or at least part of it, before job and family responsibilities would take over. My budget was only US$ 1,500. With that stack of money I bought myself an Economy class ticket to the Far East and spent the remainder on ground transportation, hotels, meals and of course souvenirs.

It took the screaming, narrow body DC-8 some 22 hours and 8 stops along the route to cover the 12,000 or so kilometers. The first few stops in this now ancient and almost extinct aircraft were exciting; Frankfurt, Rome, Athens, Dubai, Mumbai (then called Bombay). But the next stop, in the dead of night in a filthy Calcutta airport was no longer exciting. By that time all I wanted was to lie down and sleep. Fortunately the flight was not fully booked and I had three seats all to myself. So, I could stretch out and lie down more or less. In theory at least.

Unfortunately three seats were still not enough to stretch legs and my poor knees began to protest the grotesque positions I tried. The short stop in Bangkok was more interesting, simply because the entire airport smelled like teak. It must have been around 11.00 AM, but I felt as if it was in the middle of the night. My brain was asleep and my body felt battered. One more stop was scheduled in the old airport in Singapore. Nothing indicated that 20 years later Singapore would boast one of the world's best airports. Then finally we were approaching Jakarta's Kemayoran airport. With my body still fighting sleep I began to feel anxious. During the last two stretches of the flight I could no longer face the airline food and only wanted to drink. Earlier that morning the smell of omelets and coffee from the galley had made my stomach turn. The engine noise in the cabin and the whine of the air-conditioning nozzles made my head spin. On top of that came the increasing anxiety of arriving in a strange country and a strange city. Now I really began to worry. Would there be a decent taxi service in Jakarta. Would the immigration procedure be smooth? Would my bag be there, arriving on the same flight? Imagine if it had been unloaded in filthy Calcutta. All the anticipation and excitement of flying to a distant world, to see new cultures and to experience adventure had gone. It was no longer fun and I wondered what I was doing in that flying tube in the first place.

Standing in line for Immigration I felt sick, dizzy and disoriented, I could hardly stand on my feet and still felt the movements of the plane. These were the symptoms of jet lag and I would suffer from them for the next 5 days or so.

Fortunately there *was* a taxi service, although I had to haggle about the fare. The driver and his aide were dressed in rags; many of the driver's teeth were missing. They looked like plotting gangsters. The taxi itself was kept alive with the aid of strings and wire. I had serious doubts about its brakes and its engine, its tires and its everything. But at that point I couldn't care less if the driver and his aide would kidnap and kill me and rob me of my old secondhand Yashica camera and remaining US$ 500. I leaned back in the smelly seat and decided to just let it all happen. The sun was setting and the shades of green, white and many other colors were strange. I had never seen them like that. It was like I was tripping without having smoked pot. Night comes quickly in the tropics and soon everything went dark in Jakarta. Amazingly, the driver and his aide turned out to be the most sincere and helpful individuals on earth. They dropped me off at my destination with a big smile and a handshake. Even though they had had to ask directions several times and even though the trip took a lot longer than they had anticipated they hadn't asked for more money.

One week after arrival I still felt disoriented. It seemed I had no energy and had no interest in doing anything at all.

Thirty years later, after many more long and exhausting international flights, crossing countries, oceans, mountain ranges and time zones I finally mastered the art of arriving in crisp condition and going about business like nothing had happened, other than a refreshing bicycle ride to the office on a nippy morning.

Summary
In the old days flying WAS fun.

Seasickness is worse

Most long haul air travelers, even frequently flying long haul Business or First Class air travelers, arrive at their destination in a bad physical and emotional shape. With wrinkled clothes, groggy, dizzy, wobbly on the legs, feeling (and smelling) foul, and in urgent need of a bath and a bed. Even after about a week many of these air travelers still feel not fine at all. They continue to wake up in the middle of the night and by lunchtime they wish they could go to bed. These are some of the most noticeable symptoms of jet lag. And what a waste of time, productivity and fun it is.

Medical experts explain that jet lag is a condition brought about because our 'body clock' (residing in the pituitary gland, deep inside the brain –basically it's all about hormones) has difficulty keeping up with us as we speed around the globe. For example, while our eyes see that it is morning in New York, our 'body clock' signals it is time to go to bed in Europe where we were only hours ago. Even though, rationally, we agree with what our eyes see ('yes, it *is* morning'), our body or maybe our brain is serious about creating the sleepy feeling. The effects of jet lag are disorientation, sleeplessness at night, drowsiness during the day and lack of concentration. And there are many more discomforting effects your physician will be able to tell you about.

But is jet lag only the effect of a disoriented body? Maybe it also has to do with the unhealthy conditions on board a modern aircraft and the travel induced mental stress. Let's talk about the health situation first, then about stress while traveling and then you can make up your mind.

While we would associate flying with just sitting for long hours, doing next to nothing and feeling bored after awhile, air travel requires that we are physically and mentally in a good condition. We should avoid boarding our flight while we feel tired. Airline crew flying on the ultra long haul non-stop flights, during almost 20 hours are off duty four days before the flight and four days after the flight. That shows that flying is taxing our system heavily. But how many passengers can afford that luxury?

And what makes flying so taxing?
This.
The environment inside the cabin during a long flight aggravates the jet lag condition. Aircraft cabins are pressurized and noisy, air humidity is too low to be healthy and most of the air inside the cabin is filtered and circulated again and again, with only a small fraction of fresh air sucked in from outside.
Air humidity inside the aircraft is kept low to reduce the risk of corrosion of the airframe. While low humidity is good for airframes, it is not so nice for throats and bodies. Hence the suggestion in the airline's in-flight magazine to drink a lot during the journey, especially non-alcoholic drinks. Dehydration is a real risk on board commercial jets.

Despite the filtering of air a sneezing or coughing co-passenger unknowingly but liberally shares a truck-load of germs and viruses with all the other passengers and crew. A co-passenger at the other side of the cabin, suffering from TBC or SARS is capable of infecting you.
And although the cabin is pressurized, the pressure is lower than on the ground, at sea level. It is the equivalent of an altitude of some 8,ooo feet or 2,500 meters. You will not notice the difference, but your intestines do. As a result, their gas creating facility is enhanced. And that's what they happily do, those intestines of ours. They create gasses and those gasses have to get out. Ask any cabin attendant if they ever notice winding passengers. They will giggle and say 'yes, it happens all the time. You can't see it but it definitely smells.'

Fortunately airline caterers are conscious of the effects of food and digestion at high altitudes. Therefore you will not find onions, beans and such ingredients in airline food.

Cabin crews also say other things and they do so mostly among themselves and in meetings with their employers when they complain about the health hazards they endure by being exposed to the cabin climate. They urge the airlines, their employers, to improve the health condition inside the cabin by increasing the oxygen percentage. That sounds like a reasonable request. After all, without oxygen it is kind of hard to breathe. Why is it that crews have to negotiate with the airlines for a bit of fresh air? The answer is that the more oxygen is pumped inside the cabin, the more fuel it takes to do so and optimizing fuel efficiency and staying out of bankruptcy is paramount to each and every aircraft operator.

There you have it. That does not sound very encouraging. To put it briefly, to leave the aircraft in the same health condition as when you boarded it, you would need to wear an oxygen mask and also pressure stockings to keep your blood circulation going. It would be even better to wear a space suit with its own life support system. The only reason why airlines get away with their treatment of passengers is because we voluntarily agree to undergo it. We even pay for it. Or, to put it the other way, we refuse to pay three to six times more to double our living space on the aircraft or to have a bit more of oxygen. Law persons could argue that the torture therefore is self-imposed and self-inflicted. So, forget suing the airlines. And despite everything we even manage to think that flying is great and exciting. So much better than the boring daily train ride to the office. Or is it?

Flying may kill you and that is a little worse than being seasick. Yes indeed, whether you want to hear this or not, flying is dangerous. Of course there is the danger, although statistically remote, of the aircraft falling out of the sky in a steep nose-dive well before arriving at its intended destination as scheduled. Airline representatives always emphasize that traveling through the air is many times safer than crossing the street or driving your car. That is probably true. But sitting in the confined cabin space for a long time is not conducive to anybody's health. A lot has been published about DVT. No that's not the latest electronic gadget, but Deep Vein Trombosis; the clotting of the blood due to sitting for a long time in cramped conditions. Blood clots traveling from deep veins somewhere in the legs up to the brain will cause the latter to shut down. Or it may end up in the heart and stop it from beating any further. That's deadly and again, it is a lot worse than being seasick. Passengers in fact have died of DVT. In Tokyo alone 25 deaths have been linked to DVT between 1992 and 2001.

Airlines now are more proactive and offer advice on how to prevent the blood from clotting. Read about it in the in-flight magazine or watch the TV screen. Also, more and more gadgets appear on the market to stimulate the blood flow during long flights.

What those TV screens and the magazines will not tell you is that flying at high altitude increases the amount of cosmic radiation you are exposed too. Oh goodness, remember how you always carefully avoid the radiated, genetically modified food in the supermarket? And here we are on our exciting trip, finding ourselves being radiated for many hours. Admittedly, there's no need to get excited. The level of cosmic radiation is not alarming for most of us, unless you would fly long distances almost daily.

The latest discovery about long flights is pretty exciting too: jet lag causes the brain to shrink. Let's hope it's not a lasting condition and that by the time you have landed, you will remember how to get home or who those people are who meet you in the airport.

Ah, compare today's air travel hassle with those good old days of passenger ships, effortlessly plying the Atlantic in less than a week or sailing from Europe to Asian ports in about a month's time. That was the real kind of travel we (well, our grandparents) liked and that is so well suited to the physiology of the human species. Imagine yourself strolling along the deck of a luxury liner, leisurely reading for hours in a deck chair. The fresh sea breeze stirring the coiffure and the appetite. Plenty to eat and drink at no additional cost. Playing shuffleboard or chatting with one of the officers. Imagine those landfalls in strange ports with new sights and sounds and merchants vending their souvenirs.

Did you watch the film 'Titanic'? Long distance travel used to be like that, and usually without the sinking, fortunately. None of the passengers ever suffered from jet lag. At worst some might have suffered a bit from indigestion because of overeating during captain's dinners. And maybe they had to cope with seasickness.

Come to think of it seasickness may be worse than jet lag.

Anyway, pity on us who have to travel by air. Half a century ago all intercontinental travel, including air travel was a major undertaking. It was for the fur coated rich and famous, the happy few and air travel was therefore romantic. Airports were tiny and had lighthouse beacons sitting on top of the control tower to guide the pilots. The drone of propeller engines aroused sensations of excitement. Airports and aircraft handled small numbers of passengers and those individuals were catered to as very important persons. Today, air travel is nothing more than mass transportation with more and more hassle and one even wonders why some airlines still dare to advertise their service as a luxury and something that is wonderful

11

and enjoyable. Air travel is even worse than the daily train ride to the office. Praise to the Europeans who appropriately named their aircraft business Airbus. Because that's exactly what it is, an airborne bus service going from A-pore to B-town and back.

Why do we want to fly in the first place? The answer is simple. Because it is affordable. It is fast. And because there really is no feasible alternative.
So, in terms of how terrible flying is; was that all? No, unfortunately air travel is even worse than you know; it is next to a Human Rights violation. Let's see what it really is.

Summary
These days, flying is even more dangerous than driving your car.

Travel Induced Anxiety

B efore explaining what jet lag is, let's introduce its partner; please meet travel induced anxiety or just plain stress.

The question is where stress comes into the travel equation. Well, the problems with air travel basically start at home. For most of us, no matter how often we fly, the preparations of the trip come with a certain level of anxiety.

According to recent studies, many of us feel anxious about leaving home in the first place. A few days before departure we begin to feel grumpy. Interestingly, even airline pilots and experienced business travelers know the phenomenon. If at some point, you catch yourself wondering why to go on the trip, you will now know that it is an indication of pre-travel anxiety.

A different cause of this form of anxiety is that we have to be at certain places at certain points in time or else, we will miss the flight, the trip, the deal, or the expensive holiday.

Talking about missing flights, a passenger once missed his domestic flight because he had not heard the boarding announcement. Obviously it is very difficult to miss a flight once you're in the departure lounge. By the way, does departure lounge sound a bit like a euphemism for funeral parlor? It doesn't? Good, airports will be happy to hear that. Anyway, this person, who had been captivated by an article in his newspaper didn't notice the other passengers passing by, boarding the plane. He didn't read or understand the boarding sign and he had not heard that his name had been called again and again. Maybe he was too relaxed, or he simply could not hear the announcements because of the blaring TVs in the lounge and the bad quality of the PA system. After realizing, some 10 minutes later, that he had missed the flight and his important business appointment, he was very stressed, obviously. What compelling excuse would he have fabricated when he called his business partners to say he would be on the next flight? Probably something about traffic congestion on the way to the airport. The lesson is that while traveling it pays to be conscious of what goes on around us, to observe boarding announcements, and in general to be organized and focused.

Another indication of stress is boarding the wrong airplane. That is not as impossible as it seems, especially in airports where two flights board at the same time and passengers have to walk across the tarmac to the aircraft that are parked side by side.

On any trip there is an entire strain of events that induce anxiety. Even after check-in, most passengers can't relax. In these troubled times many governments impose the strictest security measures and there are airports where the definition of 'strictest' means that cabin baggage is scanned twice, that tax-free articles are carefully scrutinized for explosives or drugs and the body search makes you feel as if your next stop is the nearest high security prison. In some airports it is prudent to add another hour and sometimes even more than that in addition to the check-in time, or you might miss your flight. And then we haven't even talked about the security checks in US airports. We won't.

Traveling is waiting. It includes the waiting before boarding, the waiting before take-off, the waiting during the flight ('are we there yet?'), and then also the waiting for Immigration and Customs on arrival. No matter how fast the plane is, flying is a waiting game. All that waiting is stressful indeed.

Business travelers feel stressed as a result of the overloaded agendas they put up. The rationale is that a ticket still costs a lot of money and the more activities you cramp together while abroad the more effective and efficient the trip will be. And the more taxing it will be on your health. But auditors and accountants on average are concerned more about numbers than about passenger health.

Flying vacationers face even more stress, because of the uncertainties about their point of arrival. Will the rented car be waiting as promised? Will the hostess be there with the coach? Will the hotel exist at all? Will the pickpockets be active? Will Immigration cause problems?

Talking about Immigrations: if there would be an award for making travelers want to turn around and go home immediately Immigration Officers of quite a few countries would get it, especially those in the USA for making arriving passengers feel like criminals and Nepal for its corruption with the visa fee. In the Netherlands on the other hand one would expect the seemingly easygoing Immigration officers to invite you for a beer in the pub. In general, however, Immigration officers are not the jolliest of people.
Yet, sometimes an Immigration officer can make you smile. Stopping over in Hong Kong enroute to Xi'an, a young Immigration Officer inspected my passport for the required visas. 'Oh' he said with surprise, 'you're going to China?' 'Is this not China' I asked, only to realize then the full meaning of one country with two systems.
And sometimes an Immigration officer makes you say 'great' such as in Bangkok. A young traveler, obviously proud about his biceps and torso had dressed himself in a short and scruffy undershirt only. When it was his turn to present his passport the Immigration officer asked if he had a shirt with sleeves in his backpack and then told him to get dressed decently, if he wanted to enter the Kingdom of Thailand. That's great.

Immigration in several countries, including the holiday destination Aruba deserve an award nomination for inventing the most incomprehensible rule in the history of mankind requiring transit passengers to go through Immigration, claim their baggage, go to the

17

check-in counters and check-in for their connecting flight. Add to that the hassle of having to pay US$ 2.- for a luggage trolley, inconsistent application of the rules by Customs officers and a rude attitude of security staff, and the advice can hardly be anything else than to avoid Aruba and other similar destinations if you can.

So, next time you check in for your trip, after reading this book, you will realize that arriving in the airport two or three hours before the scheduled take-off is a complete waste of many hours of your valuable time. You could have spent those hours productively at work or happily with your family or just nervously checking your baggage and ticket and telephone numbers.
Although e-tickets, on-line check-in and self-service check-in facilities are becoming more and more main-stream, in many airports passengers still have to queue.
Standing in line at the counter for the check-in procedure you have plenty of time to ask yourself if all the paperwork is really necessary. In the 21st century is it needed to weigh each and every piece of baggage individually? Do we still need that boarding pass? Why do we still have to queue? OK, you may want to argue, but the safety regulations unfortunately need to be very tight these days and the tax-free shopping is really great. Agreed, before leaving the airport premises on board of one of those sky buses most airports really treat us on tax-free (which is not synonymous for cheap) articles. Please note that the arrival sections of airports on the other hand are very boring, sometimes even jail-like and that you're apparently expected to get out of there as soon as you can with or without damaged baggage.

No matter what, some of the pre-departure stress evaporates at the departure lounge. *Lounge*? Hah! A corral, you mean, a holding tank! There is always a shortage of seats and often an excess of noise in those 'lounges'. You always have to wait there for too long.

Children play, cry or scream because the waiting bores them. Several TV sets are blaring different programs simultaneously. The PA system announces a delay, a gate change or tells us to remain seated because women and children will board first. As if the airport is going to sink, while in fact only Osaka's Kansai airport is known to sink. All the others don't, including Amsterdam's Schiphol airport that is situated some 5 meters below sea level.

Airlines could make their passengers happier by adopting a different approach to boarding. Instead of holding everyone in the corral, why not complete the preparations (cleaning, catering) inside the aircraft earlier and allow passengers to board one by one after clearing the final security check. It would certainly make congestion and pushing at the gate a thing of the past. Inside the aircraft it would also do away with the waiting in the aisles when passengers try to store their carry-on baggage.

Anyway, once you are boarding the aircraft and after more hassle and pushing and being hit by oversized cabin luggage of co-passengers who urgently want to pass you in the aisle, you will find yourself in your economy class seat. Seat? Sitting device or containing frame would be a more appropriate name. Did you notice that the airline has generously allowed you less than half a square meter to live your life for the next 3 or 6 or 15 hours? In the comfort of your own home, try to sit in your most comfortable chair for one hour. Don't even get up to go to the kitchen. Just sit there for one hour. Chances are that you will not be able to remain in your chair for more than 15 minutes. It's just not natural to be immobile for an extended period. To make things worse, in the aircraft cabin up to two more individuals are assigned similar containing frames next to yours, boxing you in even more if you are unlucky enough to get the middle seat. Of course, although you have no say in the selection of who will be packed next to you, unconsciously you expect the beautiful woman or the handsome young businessman from the airline ad to sit next to you.

Did you notice that airlines always brag about the niceties of their first and business classes? They hardly ever say anything about their cattle class (also dubbed; economy or coach class). Brace yourself because instead of the slick and refined individuals from the ad, it could very well be an oversized person, badly smelling or badly mannered. This person may immediately colonize the armrest, open a newspaper, leaving you even less space for *your* aura.

About armrests, please note that airlines in their attempts to optimize the use of space in the cabin provide every three Economy Class passengers (having six elbows) only four armrests. Psychologists could design an interesting study on how the sharing of the armrests occurs. Never have I witnessed passengers discussing the subject. Usually it's a matter of body language and eye contact avoidance. The most dominant passenger simply puts his or her arms squarely and convincingly on the rests, even if the other passenger or passengers were seated there before. If the other passengers are less dominant they will give in quickly, removing their elbow, thus accepting even less space. Since I became aware of what was happening I like to put up a bit of a fight, leaving my arms on the rest, making sure that my elbow touches the dominant person's elbow. I even poke the challenger's elbow while I pretend to fumble with the in-flight magazine. Sometimes that helps.

There is a bit more to share about the armrest. It's amazing that the manufacturers of airline seats have made a science out of designing a comfortable seat that even holds in-flight entertainment gadgets, but that they always overlook the comfort rate of the armrest. Take another look; the armrest is lined with aluminum or hard plastic. It is tough and on a long flight eventually your arms don't want to rest themselves there at all. It may be just a matter of time until a passenger sues an airline for causing 'armrest elbow' –that's something similar to a tennis elbow.

In a little while we'll see that to prevent jet lag sleep and relaxation during the flight are essential. You may ask "How can I possibly sleep with so much noise around me, sitting in such a cramped position and with such armrests?!"
Rest assured it can be done. It's all a matter of disciplining or conditioning yourself. After awhile you may even begin to feel drowsy whenever you approach an airport.

But of course, for now you will primarily remember those previous flights when your sight was blocked by your neighbor's newspaper, your nose was offended by armpit odor, while your ears were bombarded by the air conditioning and engine sounds, and on top of everything, your armrests colonized. You are right, as soon as the 'fasten seatbelts' sign goes off many passengers get up and begin to move around the cabin, looking for some personal space. Ah, and then to make things even more interesting the passenger in front of you decides to use all the technical features of the seat, fully reclining its backrest. Each time that happens to me I get really cross (as the Brits say politely). Fully reclining the seat in Economy Class borders on an act of violence. It's mere aggression. It is a human rights violation, an intrusion into one's private space, or what's left of it. It is nothing else but an anti-social act and all airlines should be held responsible for committing such intolerable acts. An innovative little gadget is on the market now that allows a passenger to block the seat in front from fully reclining. Some airlines allow it, others have outlawed its use, arguing that all passengers have the right to recline their seats. Which seems to imply that other passengers don't have the right to breathe.

So, if you had planned to open your laptop and work a bit during the long flight in Economy class, now is the time to forget all about it. You're a sardine in a can and canned sardines are not supposed to move or do laptop work. Meanwhile, your oversized neighbor, having returned from a first stroll to the toilet and having read the newspaper, drops all the pages on the floor and decides it is time for a beer. You don't know it yet, but he will be drinking beer all flight long, adding another smell to the variety you have to cope with already. He hurts your legs and knees each time he tries to stumble in front of you on his way to and from the toilet to discharge the excess beer.
That is the opposite of relaxation during the flight.
And then, during night flights when you begin to feel tired there always seems to be a group of holiday-makers to keep you awake. They are so excited that they chat and laugh all night long, playing cards, loudly but unknowingly creating their jet lag.

Is that the romance of subsonic air travel? No, on the contrary, it's stress, stress, and more stress. No wonder that you confuse your body by exposing it to such torture.

And yet, it is very well possible to make the trip bearable. A small contribution to a nicer flight has to do with tidiness. Sooner or later, it is your turn to get up from your seat and move past other passengers, lining up in front of the toilets. When you do so you must be careful for the mess passengers are creating in the cabin. Why is it that western countries (and Singapore) look so clean? It is because of a very efficient waste collecting system and strict law enforcement. In the absence of those, like in aircraft cabins you will see that humankind is filthy. Newspapers, headset bags, blanket wrappings, breadcrumbs and a few plastic cups litter the floor under the seats and these can and every now and then do make it to the aisles, creating a risk for you and others to slip and fall. I once saw that happen to a cabin attendant. And it's not any better in business or first class.

Ah, we haven't complained yet about infants on board. Should we? Many passengers give up hope of a quiet flight when they see infants being carried on board. But in fact, infants are the quietest passengers. They may cry or scream, but usually that is only before take off. Once airborne, they go asleep and wake up only when it is feeding time or nappy changing time. Who knows, the cabin noise may remind them of the familiar sounds when still inside their mother's womb.

Talking about screaming. Many airlines are increasingly worried about 'passenger craze' or passengers behaving out of control, screaming and yelling, threatening to open the door or to physically assault the crew or other passengers. Behavior analysts and cabin crews say that excessive alcohol use and pre-boarding frustrations are at the root of this growing problem. Passenger craze costs airlines millions of dollars every year. The analysts are probably right: it's all about travel induced stress. Hence, with airports getting more crowded by the hour, security screenings that border on the intolerable and indecent, and air travel suffering delays more and more, passenger craze is probably here to stay. One airline once suggested limiting the use of alcohol to two servings per passenger. Great, how would they control that? By putting a stamp on passengers' foreheads after each drink, maybe?

Yes, passenger craze is indeed a problem. Maybe it is triggered when someone reclines the seat or colonizes an armrest.
Not always does passenger craze come with screaming and violence. On one homeward bound flight a couple refused to take their seats; unhappy as they were that

their seats were in the last row of the plane. They remained standing, even when the plane was pushed back from the gate. The engines were started and they still didn't sit down. Eventually the plane had to return to the gate to allow security personnel to take the unwilling passengers into custody and off the flight.

Fortunately, more and more air passengers and air passenger associations are demanding better economy classes at affordable rates. Almost all airlines have implemented some improvements. At least they have created an 'uptown' economy class with better seats, usually called Premium Class. Of course it is more expensive than the regular Economy Class. There you have it, this is the proof: airlines know that Economy Class is bad. With that, the creation of an improved class between Business and Economy reduces the latter even more to Third Class. One airline has adopted a different approach, creating a Basic class, which is cheaper than Economy and with fewer services still. Confusing, isn't it?

Summary:
There is always hope.

Homesickness

R elated to travel induced anxiety or stress is feeling homesick. Why is homesickness never discussed in travel literature? It must be very real on many occasions for many of us, and that includes seasoned business travelers as well.

Yes, travel to faraway places on the other side of the globe will make some of those who don't have to travel envy you. They find it difficult to believe that travel is not just fun and happy hour all the time wherever you are.

Unless they travel for a few weeks themselves they won't understand that feeling homesick is often part of the travel game.

Vacationers likewise run the risk of a partly spoilt vacation trip when they get homesick. The risk of a wasted vacation because of homesickness is very real. Having spent several years organizing tours through South East Asia I learned that homesickness usually sets in after one or two weeks into the trip. The strange surroundings with all those unfamiliar sights, sounds, and smells can become too overwhelming. Communication barriers begin to take their toll sooner or later and all that the traveler wants is to go home.

A tourist in Indonesia, half way through his tour arrived in the enticing city of Jogjakarta. He was not very happy with the hotel and his already not so happy mood worsened. One morning during breakfast he suddenly exploded. Yelling at the scared staff he demanded ham and bacon. His poor and embarrassed wife could not calm him down and he didn't want to hear or accept the explanation that in this largely Muslim environment ham and bacon simply are not available. This was a different kind of passenger craze or guest craze, safely on the ground.

As a young travel agent I once made a long trip to Japan, Hong Kong and Thailand. The trip was expensive for our small travel agency. It was a big investment and I had been looking forward to it for quite a while. On the day of departure my wife and baby daughter saw me off at the airport and, lo and behold, I found it hard to say goodbye. My daughter called me when I went through Immigration. I imagined my wife, having to do all the chores all by herself and taking care of the baby as well. Would she manage? The voice of my daughter still sounded in my ears. I missed her. All of that kept lingering in my mind and made me feel homesick even before I boarded the aircraft. All in all I didn't enjoy the trip very much. It turned into a waste of money, simply because I could not focus on the job enough.

The learning for me was to forget about home for the duration of the trip. Making telephone calls or sending e-mail is fine, but by all means, leave the problems of home at home. The loved ones can take care of themselves. And if they can't, don't leave home without them.

Summary:
When traveling, leave home at home and focus on the task at hand.

Jet Lag: what it is

A s we revealed earlier, experts explain that jet lag is caused because our body (they say 'body clock') still follows time in the time zone where we use to live or where we have spent the last few weeks, while the body (that's us) has been jetted to a different place several time zones away. The body simply lags behind in catching up to the new time zone. Poor body for not knowing what is happening. We should have told it. And so we will.

For most individuals it is not a problem to cross up to three time zones, but crossing more than four is almost certainly asking for a confused body, it's asking for jet lag. A lot has been said, discussed and researched about jet lag. If you're interested in more scientifically profound theories about the phenomenon, search "jet lag" or "jetlag" or even "jet-lag" on the Web and you will find a number of sites with varying degrees of scientific explanations (also see the last page of this book for some of these sites).

Scientists agree that modern air travel causes a disturbance in our sleep rhythm or circadian rhythm. They say that for every hour of time difference, the body needs one day to recover. The math is easy: if your trip takes you across 10 time zones, you will need 10 days to become the usual you again. That's a long time for a, let's say, five day trip.

There are many different approaches to treating jet lag. They may include such things as light therapy, diets, meditation and acupuncture. Allopathic and homeo-pathic drugs, developed to avoid the modern air traveler from feeling groggy on arrival, are available too, but some of them don't work or they have serious side effects, doctors warn. Most of these drugs contain melatonin, the hormone produced by the pineal gland, which regulates our wake-sleep rhythm. The natural production of melatonin increases when daylight decreases and night falls. As a result we begin to feel sleepy. Some research results indicate that melatonin can best be taken after arrival, rather than before or during the flight. Melatonin should not be used without a prescription, even though in several countries it is available as an over-the-counter drug. So, be careful if you decide to use a chemical anti-jet lag drug.

Some air passengers try to adjust to the time zone at their destination in a more natural way. A few days before departure they simply shift their wake-sleep pattern by adjusting the times they get up in the morning and go to bed at night. That is not such a bad idea, if it were not for the practical complications it causes. For a time difference of up to four hours it is doable, but once the traveler has to cross 12 time zones it gets rather more complicated. Inviting guests for tea at three in the morning may raise an eyebrow or two.

In this book we'll forget all about melatonin and other drugs and explain how you can adjust your body clock in a different way, without having to go to work in the middle of the night.

Let's go back to the basics: a slow body clock.
Essentially, that's all what jet lag is about. But it is also very much influenced by a confused and stressed mind as we discussed earlier. Now we need to know if we can avoid it. The answer fortunately is affirmative. Yes, we can successfully avoid jet lag or at least significantly reduce its effects. The theory behind the positive answer is amazingly simple: like we can adjust any clock or watch, so can we adjust our body clock. The way to prevent jet lag, propagated through these pages is through mentally talking to yourself. Call it self-hypnosis or meditation or anything else; all you need to do is to tell your body and your mind what is going to happen during the long journey and to follow a very simple procedure.

To be fully free from jet lag may require several long haul flights, but you should at least notice a positive difference even after your first flight if you follow the simple procedure explained in the next chapter.

Summary

While traveling, adjust all clocks.

Preventing Jet Lag

S o, we now have demystified modern air travel. Have I exaggerated about the health and stress situation when flying? Airline officials will say I have. Passenger activists will say I haven't gone far enough.

Whatever the case may be, while trying to prevent jet lag it doesn't hurt to work from a worst-case scenario. Keep your expectations low to reduce the opportunities for disappointment and frustration and to increase opportunities to enjoy the trip and to arrive in ship shape condition, ready to make holiday or to do business. So, have a plan B ready in case you discover that your flight reservation can nowhere be found in the computer, or that you will arrive at your destination three days late. Before leaving home it is best to assume that your flight will be fully booked, that you will end up in a middle seat in the middle row in the back of the plane and that there will be delays. Also assume that one of your suitcases will take a different flight in an opposite direction and that you may never see it again (although in reality luggage retrieval is rather sophisticated and effective in this day and age).

Having said all that, let's not dwell on the theory of avoiding jet lag (basically I haven't any), but see how the avoiding works. As we said before, no drugs are needed, unless you have a headache on your trip.

Let's see if we can make a virtual intercontinental flight of 15 hours, covering 6 time zones. We will fly east, which many travelers say is the most difficult direction in terms of coping with jet lag. Our virtual flight is scheduled to leave around 20.00 hours (08.00 PM) –in the aviation industry times are always expressed in the 24 hour, or military format. After that we'll discuss how to deal with other and longer flights both east and to the west.

Now, watch this. Leaving today at 8 in the evening and flying east means that we will arrive at our destination around 17.00 hours (05.00 PM) tomorrow. That will be well after local teatime. It will be happy hour with dinnertime approaching. However, according to your body clock it will be only 11.00 hours (11.00 AM) at home after a night with lots of noise and little sleep. Your body will be in the mood for another strong cup of coffee, but with only a few hours of sleep, more than anything else it will be asking for a bed, a soft pillow and a quiet room. You will feel exhausted and very lousy. Let's try to avoid the lousy feeling and the craving for a bed.

It all starts with good preparations for your long trip across the globe. Here we go.

Making your reservation

Every flight begins with a reservation. If you're a frequent flyer you probably will have a frequent flyer pass that entitles you to certain benefits. One of those may be the right to request a certain seat in a certain part of the aircraft. The best seats in the aircraft are on the flight deck. However these are taken. There are still other seats in the front of the cabin and these are for passengers paying a lot of money for Business or First Class or Economy Premium –all depending on the type of aircraft and its configuration. Our challenge, as Economy class passengers is to get a seat as far in the front section of the cabin as possible. There, ahead of the engines the noise is not as disturbing as further aft. Some airlines will allow us to request a certain seat but they will not confirm it.

There is more to seats than just requesting one in front. On our long flight to the east with 50 percent of it during the night we need to decide if a window seat will be nice or an aisle seat. The latter gives you more freedom to get up and go to the toilet without disturbing others. On wide body aircraft there are far more aisle seats than window seats. But a window seat offers you at least one armrest without having to fight for it. And the window, even in the middle of the night gives wonderful sights of a seemingly peaceful world below.

Tall passengers like to try and find a seat with a lot of legroom. The front row seats are favorite among them, but only the front row seats identified with B, C, H and J near one of the doors offer the sought after legroom. In the other front row seats (usually identified with A, D, E, F, and G) you will likely face a bulkhead and there you have even less space for your legs than in a regular seat. Smaller aircraft like the Boeing 737 series have more space than average near one of the emergency exits, but the disadvantage of those seats is that the backrest does not recline. But then again, Boeing 737s never make long haul flights.

Still about making preparations for your trip, one of the options you have when making a booking is to order a special meal. Most airlines have more than the regular meal that comes out of the trolley. If you are a vegetarian, you will be happy to know that there are several vegetarian meals to choose from. There are also kosher meals, Hindu meals and Moslem meals. Airlines even offer gluten free meals, no sodium meals and meals for diabetics. Probably the most unknown meal options are seafood meal and fresh fruit platter. The fresh fruit platter is great when you have to fly half way or further across the globe. Fruit platters are light and easy to digest.

Ask your travel agent or the airline for the full range of meal options. Don't ask for special meals when you check in or are already on board, but at the time you make your reservations.

The fun of a special meal is that they are usually served ahead of the pack. The drawback is that the empty tray will be cleared only with the clearing of the pack's empty trays. That means that you will sit with litter in front of you a little longer than your fellow passengers will.

Preparations at home

Ask the travel agent for a timetable of the airline(s) you will use or look them up through the airlines' websites. In the timetables there is a section that spells out the meal services for each flight, the duration of the flights and the stopover points. If you have time to study all those details it's great reading to bring you in the proper travel mood and it is excellent learning. These data help you in planning to avoid jet lag too.

So, here's the first part of the anti jet lag secret. Avoiding jet lag begins at home, before you go to the airport. If you are a busy business traveler, working until it is almost too late to leave for the airport, the same principle still applies. Begin preparing your body (and your mind) while you work. It is not a big thing; you can even do it while chairing a last minute meeting.

Even so, it is best to have a few hours of nothing else to do than to check your passport, money or credit cards and the tickets. You may want to make a last minute call to the airline (not the travel agent) checking if your flight is still scheduled to leave on time. Having done that it is time to get a shower, to shave (female travelers may skip this part) and to change into your most comfortable travel outfit. Forget about the jacket, the new shining shoes, the necktie, the high heels and the expensive hairdo. For female travelers, accessories and jewelry may make you feel uncomfortable. Remember; traveling these days has nothing to do with the glamour of the early years of flight in the first half of the 20th century. It's just a simple bus ride.

Maximizing relaxation and comfort, rather then appearance is all that matters. The shower and the changing of clothes are meant to tell your body that it will be bedtime early today. Assuming that you shave only once every 24 hours as part of your waking up ritual, the shaving will ensure that you arrive at your destination without a disturbing roughness at the chin and cheeks.

Nobody ever talks about it. However, now that we have admitted that travel comes with a certain amount of anxiety, we also need to talk about toilets. Toilet use between the time you are still at home right until the moment you board the aircraft needs to be managed. You probably will need 'to go' more often than on a regular day at work. So, manage toilet use if you can.

And don't leave for the airport at the very last minute. Remember you still have a seat to confirm and checking in early may do the trick. The traffic to the airport will probably be jammed. The train will probably be delayed for no apparent reason. All the other enroute-to-the-airport things will probably also not go smooth. Since you are trying to avoid jet lag and since that comes with feeling relaxed you will not do yourself a favor by being almost late or too late for all the required procedures.

Traveling light
Many airlines try to strictly enforce the rules that limit the number of pieces of cabin baggage passengers can carry into the cabin. That makes a lot of sense when you see what passengers try to lug around as 'cabin baggage'. Basically everything that is in excess of the checked baggage allowance is going to be 'cabin baggage' these passengers reason. That explains the common sight of people struggling with two or three really big and heavy

bags, in addition to a trolley case and a sizeable cardboard box. Don't be amazed if this much 'carry on' stuff weighs in at another 20 kilograms (some 40 pounds) or more per person. Handling all those kilograms or pounds is anything but relaxing. It is also not very civilized to fellow passengers to occupy so much space in the overhead lockers. The message is clear: travel as light as you can. An overnight bag or a small carry-on trolley holds a lot of stuff. If you're a tax-free shopper it is smart to leave some room in that bag, sufficient to hold the tax-free articles you think you will not be able to resist.

Be critical about the things you need to bring with you. Usually it is a lot less than you assume.

In the airport

Checking in usually is one of the most hassle free parts of the entire journey, providing you don't show up at the counter with excess baggage or at the very last minute. Staff are friendly and want to hand you the boarding pass as quickly as they can. Don't forget to ask about your favorite seat or if your meal choice has been confirmed. If it cannot be confirmed, no problem. Since you had no expectations you also had no hopes of getting either one, and so you will not lose your temper or feel disappointed. Simply ask for a similar seat as much forward as possible and ask if they can still do something about the meal. On long flights avoid the middle seats!

More and more airlines use e-tickets and Internet check-in, while airports offer self-service check-in points. These are positive developments. They reduce queuing and save you time.

Boarding and Departure (Flying east)

By the time you go through customs you need to communicate with your body. It will now be around 19.00 hours (7 PM), early evening and there's almost an hour left before take off. Now it is really time to let everything go. Tell your body accordingly. Feel relaxed, you're going on a long trip and it will be enjoyable. That's the message you need to convince your body and mind of. Here are some ingredients to help you with the convincing. Obviously you feel great after your afternoon shower and shave. There is still plenty of time to do some shopping. Treat yourself on something: a special magazine, a chocolate bar, anything that is enjoyable to you. Approaching the holding tank (remember it is referred to as waiting lounge or gate), it will be crowded outside. In most airports the departure lounges are opened only half an hour before boarding time. It is now important to position yourself strategically so that, when the passengers are allowed to enter the area you don't have to stand in line too long. You may want to resist the temptation to sit down –after all you can do so for the next 15 hours. After the final cabin baggage check and the checking with the metal detector walk straight to near the gate doors. The objective is to enter the aircraft first or as early as possible to avoid all the pushing that comes when the crowds go inside.

Most airlines allow elderly and handicapped passengers and passengers with children to board first. First class, business class passengers and holders of elite frequent flyer passes may board as they please and will also be among the first to go aboard. Some airlines then board by row number; some others just allow the hoard to squeeze through the gate and into the aircraft. Either way it is easy to board as one of the first passengers –if you know how to do it. Boarding early is nice because you will not have to search for space in the overhead lockers.

Call it meditation or self-hypnosis or whatever you

like; now comes the most important point of the entire journey. Once seated, tell your body that here is where you will live for the next 15 hours and that you are going to make the most of it.

Please check and make sure: half a square meter of space is all you will have at your disposal. A jail cell is more spacious. Anyway, jail cells don't fly to exciting destinations, so let's cope with our 0.5 m² without complaining. Before buckling up, make sure you have all the necessities for the night ready. And this is another secret to prevent jet lag: it is essential to catch as much sleep as possible. With all the noise and people talking and walking around that is not so simple. Therefore you need a few gadgets to dress for the night (try them at home first to check if they are comfortable):

- Eyeshades
- Earplugs or noise canceling headset
- An inflatable pillow

These three pieces of equipment are very important. If you like you may bring some optional stuff such as:

- A bottle of water to take a sip in the middle of the night without the need to get up from your seat,
- Prescription medicines as needed,
- A few aspirins may be effective in preventing, blood clots, because they make the blood thinner
- You may like to wear a watch that shows the time in two different locations, although the time at your destination is also available from the flight monitoring system in the cabin
- The newly bought magazine or chocolate bar

For the time being just put it all in the seat pocket

in front of you. Make yourself comfortable and make your body understand, in a positive 'tone' that you are going to sit for the next so many hours. Although sleep is usually associated with lying down, tonight you will sleep while seated.

It is time to kick off your shoes, to buckle up and to enjoy seeing passengers searching for their seats, struggling with their carry-on luggage, scrambling to put it all in the overhead bins. Yeah, when passengers try to pass each other in the aisles then you know that aisles are narrow and designed only for narrow trolleys and young and slender cabin attendants pushing those trolleys.

OK, once we're all there and the doors are closed it's time for take off. Relax, this is fun.

In flight, after take-off:

As soon as the 'fasten seatbelt' sign goes off, passengers will begin to walk. You will not, for the simple reason that cabin attendants at the same time also get up and begin to serve drinks, peanuts, headsets and blankets. It's peak hour for them and like all good passengers do, please make their life and their job easier by quietly sitting down.

One alcoholic drink with the peanuts and another one for dinner should not be a problem. After all, you are enjoying yourself. But not more than two drinks! Dinner will be served roughly an hour and a half after take off or around 21.30 (09.30 PM). After the dinner you can enjoy the after dinner entertainment, either the in-flight entertainment or the magazine you bought in the airport. Take care to keep the environment clean. Headset wrappings make great waste bags.

Around your regular at home bedtime you will need to begin prepare for the night. This is an important part of the entire trip and critical in preventing jet lag. No need to change into your bed gown or to brush your teeth. The eyeshades, earplugs and pillow will do. If the pillow provided by the airline is comfortable, by all means use it making sure that it supports the back of your neck so that your head does not roll sideways. Good earplugs will reduce the sound pollution significantly, especially the high pitch noises. A nice high tech earplug comes in the shape of a noise reduction headset that generates its own anti-sound, a frequency opposite to that of the frequency generated by the air conditioning and the engines. The result is not perfect silence, but the sound reduction is rather acceptable. These headsets come at a price of roughly US$ 50 and up. You'll find them in more and more airports and electronics stores.

The eyeshades ensure that the flickering of the film screen, the cabin lights or the reading lights of other passengers will not disturb you. Now, all there is left to do is to assume a relaxing upright sleeping position and to tell your body to go to sleep.

Surprising as it may sound, the most relaxing position to sleep while sitting is by sitting upright. Some passengers are master sleepers. They simply pull the blanket over their heads, curl up somehow and they're off until someone wakes them up after the landing. Others are not so fortunate. Some will lean forward trying to rest their heads against the seat in front of them. That puts a lot of strain on the forehead, the neck and the stomach and usually is not comfortable for more than two minutes. Then they try to sleep resting on their left or right side. Wrong again, backs and shoulders, the spleen and the other intestines don't like those positions. So, the best position to sleep during the flight is by sitting straight. It is not even required or recommended to fully recline the seat. Test a few positions to find out which one puts the least stress on your buttocks while still supporting the lower part of your back and the back of your neck.

You also have to find a place for your arms. Folding them across the chest is not comfortable after a while, neither resting them on the armrest. Here the tray table comes to the rescue. It is big enough to use as an armrest; try it.

The last critical thing to do before dozing off is adjusting your watch to the time at the destination. From now on forget everything about the time at your origin. Focus on the destination.

Good night and sweet dreams. With a bit of luck you'll manage five or six hours of sleep, even if it feels like you can't sleep at all. The point is not to worry. You'll probably wake up briefly now and then to adjust your legs and feet or to take a sip of water.

You'll probably wake up while the aircraft cabin is still dark. Looking at your watch you'll be happy to see that at your destination it is already late morning. Great, waking up in the morning is what people are designed for. Cabin attendants want us to keep the window shades down to create the effect of night until *they* are ready to begin serving breakfast, but there's no need for you to go with that show. Ignore the darkness of the cabin, ignore the snoring of other passengers. Feel the morning! Morning is morning and mornings are fine. By now the cabin, with the exception of your half a meter of living space is a real mess as you'll notice while you get up and go to the toilet to brush your teeth. See, the mirror confirms that what you look at is a face of an energized person waking up in the morning while birds are singing in the trees (36,000 feet or more below). With most passengers still asleep and before the cabin crew begins to work you have time to stretch your legs and to try the exercises that the airline suggests in its in-flight magazine to get the blood streams flowing.

The rest of the flight is peanuts. It comes with all the routine daily stuff, like having breakfast, some reading or a bit of work and listening to music and watching a movie. Check your watch regularly and the position of the sun (or alternatively the shadows it makes in the clouds) to make sure that your body realizes that the short morning is changing to afternoon. That is one of the other important moments; you need to be aware of the differences, especially the different atmosphere between your regular mornings and afternoons at home or at work and then consciously switch from morning feeling to afternoon feeling, without protesting that the morning has been too short. We'll make up for that on the way home. Sounds silly, but it is very effective. Mornings and afternoons come with different shades of lights and those are plentiful outside the aircraft, so open the window shade and enjoy the view.

On arrival

Approximately an hour and a half to two hours after landing and going through all the excitement of Immigration, collecting bags and checking Customs you will be home or in your hotel. It is early evening and time for a bite if you feel like it. Still, overeating needs to be avoided because your system requires time to settle down.

Although you may feel a bit drowsy don't go to bed until it is your usual bedtime or a little earlier than that. Leave the curtains open so that your 'body clock' will quickly respond to the sunrise the following morning. Then, waking up, you'll be as crisp as usual, ready for work or to enjoy the holiday.

Your Jet Lag is a thing of the past!

This was an easy to handle mere fifteen-hour flight.

For longer flights the same principles in avoiding jet lag apply, but the result may not be optimal. The cause simply is the health unfriendly cabin environment as we discussed before. Therefore, on trips spanning more than 6 or 7 time zones it is best to make an overnight stop. A two-day stop is even better before continuing to your final destination.

If you have to go on a very long business trip with a flight of more than 15 hours and your employer does not allow you a stopover, produce some of the compelling health advice on making long flights and make a point of being allowed a stopover.

Flying west

Flying west (the opposite direction of the previous virtual flight) requires the same principles to avoid jet lag. Let's briefly point out the highlights of a 15-hour night flight in the opposite direction of the flight we have discussed in detail. We are going to fly from Jakarta to Amsterdam via Singapore.

Pre-departure preparations consist of taking a shower and shaving. Change into your most comfortable travel outfit. Be on time for everything.

In-flight preparations are outlined below.

Jakarta to Singapore, flight time: 1 hour 15 minutes

Jet lag prevention:

Departure from Jakarta is 19.00 hours (07.00 PM). The flight from Jakarta to Singapore is brief and you can take it easy. The time difference between Jakarta and Singapore is one hour and that makes the arrival time 21.15 (09.15 PM). No need to set your watch yet. Just enjoy the short ride. The stopover in Singapore will be approximately one hour and passengers will have the opportunity to browse and shop in the tax-free section of Changi airport and enjoy all the excellent facilities there.

Time flies so don't be late for boarding. For safety reasons the plane will not leave without you, but it is not nice to be the last passenger to board the aircraft, especially if your name has been called several times.

Singapore to Amsterdam, flight time 13 hours

Jet lag prevention:
OK, this is it. Take off time is 22.30 (10.30 PM). With the serving of peanuts and the snack it will be past midnight when dinner is served. Be careful with late dinners. Don't eat it all if you're not starving. By the time the leftovers are cleared it will be around 01.00 in the early hours of the morning. Don't panic about too short a night to catch some sleep. Now it is time to set your watch to the time at your destination. Then you will see that it is still 18.00 (06.00 PM) there. That's early dinnertime. Or it will be 17.00 (05.00 PM) if you fly during European daylight saving time –happy hour. See, no need to worry about staying up late. Even though it is dark outside in Asia, you can still make yourself feel the late afternoon or early evening atmosphere you are used to at home. With a remaining flying time of more than 10 hours there is still plenty of time to catch a good amount of sleep. By the time the feature movie starts and the cabin is still full of chatter and passengers and crew moving back and forth, you go through the routine of getting 'dressed' for the night. Earplugs, eyeshades, bottle of water, comfortable position. Pull the shades over your eyes or put the blanket over your head and then it is 'lights off' for the next 6 hours. Sweet dreams.

If you have got the hang of sleeping on board a jet, roaring though the skies at 850 up to 1,000 Km per hour you will wake up some two or three hours before landing. The flight monitoring system will tell you that you are somewhere in Central Europe. And in case you wake up while breakfast is being served you will know that you sort of overslept. Now, that's a new concept in air travel!

Touching down very early in the morning, around 06.00, contrary to many of your co-passengers you feel refreshed. It's time for a shave (if you're an adult male passenger) and a shower. You will be able to enjoy those luxuries around 08.00 in your hotel or at home. See, exactly what you always do in the morning.

The rest of the day is easy. If you feel sleepy before lunchtime you should treat yourself to a nap. Don't sleep long, though. Set your alarm clock to wake you up after not more than two hours. Then, at night go to bed at your usual time or a little earlier. Leave the curtains open so your body will respond to daybreak.

Summary: To prevent jet lag focus on your destination.

More Practice Flights

M ore flight examples with long and short flights, flying east and flying west will help to make you comfortable with the simple principle of avoiding jet lag, which is to focus on your destination.

First of all we'll have a look at a short and easy 8 hour flight from Frankfurt (FRA) to New York's John F. Kennedy International (JFK), crossing 7 time zones.

From FRA to JFK, flight time 8 hours (a direct flight)

Jet lag prevention:

Departure time 11.40 (11.40 AM). Flying time a little more than 8 hours, arrival in New York 18.30 (06.30 PM).

You will cover 6 time zones in 8 hours. This westward daytime flight seems deceivingly easy, but is long enough to cause a solid jet lag.

Remember to set your watch to the time in New York early in the flight. In New York at that time, the traffic is still quiet in anticipation of the morning rush hour. The Europe to East Coast, USA flights are great to work or to read a lot. Or to watch two movies. But don't overdo it. Sometime after lunch, take a nap of two hours.

On arrival in New York it will be rush hour –office workers are going home in throngs.

By the time you arrive home or in your hotel it will be around 8 or 9 in the evening. Time for a shower and then, without much ado, go to sleep.

And now a 10 hours flight from Tokyo (TYO) to Los Angeles (LAX), passing the International Date Line, spanning 8 time zones.

TYO to LAX, flight time: 10 hours

Previously you may have looked at a 10 hour flight as

something boring. But now, the problem is that this flight may not be long enough to allow you to enjoy five or six hours of well deserved sleep!

Jet lag prevention: Take off from Tokyo's Narita airport is scheduled for 17.20 (05.20 PM). The Jumbo Jet, a Boeing 747-400 or Boeing 777 will not make any stops (there's only sea down below) and fly you all the way to Los Angeles International in a little less than 10 hours. On take off, set your watch to LA time and convince body and mind of the time at your destination. Then have dinner and watch a bit of movie. Don't stay up too long, or you will not get your 6 hours of sleep.
When you wake up, the cabin crew may already be busy with the breakfast. Open the window shade and let in the morning feeling.
On arrival in LA you will probably feel very ready to do business, but it is better to take it easy. Take a nap after lunchtime; not more than two hours and, in the evening, go to bed early. Leave the curtains open to let in the first daylight the next morning.

That went well, so how about an 11.5 hours flight from Los Angeles (LAX) to Tokyo (TYO), flying west and passing the International Date Line, arriving the same day

LAX to TYO, flight time 11 hours, 20 minutes
Jet lag prevention:
Departure from Los Angeles International is set for 13.00 (01.00 PM), arrival 16.20 (04.20 PM). This should be a nice flight, providing turbulence across the Pacific is not too bad. It should be a great flight, since you can catch up on sleep. Take it easy, the day will be long. You will have plenty of time to read or work, to enjoy the meal service and the in-flight entertainment. Don't forget to set your watch to Tokyo time. After

some 7 hours in flight, close your eyes for a very long afternoon nap. Wake up around 14.00 (02.00 PM) Tokyo time.

At your destination stay up until around 21.00 (09.00 PM).

OK, those were the easy flights. Now we go for the more serious stuff. Let's have a try at a more than 20 hours trip from London Heathrow (LHR) to Sydney (SYD) flying east through Bangkok (BKK). You will experience short nights, arriving after two days and 11 time zones!

LHR to SYD. First leg: LHR to BKK, flight time 11 hours, 30 minutes

Jet lag prevention:

Less then 12 hours in the air. Should be peanuts by now. Departure from Heathrow is 22.30 (10.30 PM), arrival in Bangkok is 16.05 (04.15 PM) the next day. Anti jet lag preparations are similar to the first flight we discussed. Set your watch to Bangkok time shortly before going to sleep. Likewise the challenge during this night flight is to make you experience the change from morning to late afternoon in a very brief time span.

Second leg: BKK to SYD flight time 7 hours, 40 minutes

Jet lag prevention:

Little time in Bangkok's International airport to stretch your legs. Tax-free articles are plentiful, varied and of good quality but generally quite expensive. The waiting sections at the gates are most boring and depressing. It's a good thing that the construction of a brand new airport is in progress.

Your flight continues at 17.40 (05.40 PM), arriving the next day at 05.20 (05.20 AM). Set your watch to Sydney time. Will you be up to another 4 or 5 hours of sleep? Try it after some 3 hours in flight and don't worry if you wake up after only 2 or 3 hours. The good thing about waking up early, before breakfast is served is that you won't have to queue to get to the toilet.

On arrival it's time for a long shower and afterwards to take it easy for the rest of the day. A nap of one or two hours around 11 o'clock the same morning is perfectly fine and a siesta of the same duration is good also. Go to bed early, leaving the curtains open to catch the first morning light the following day.

Another long flight is this 24 hours and 23 minutes trip from Melbourne (MEL) in Australia, all the way to Chicago, Illinois, USA (ORD) with a stop in Auckland, New Zealand (AKL). You will cross 10 time zones.

MEL to ORD. First stretch: MEL to AKL, flight time 3 hours, 15 minutes

Jet lag prevention:

24 hours in the air! If you like to try this trip in one go, without taking a good night's sleep in Los Angeles, please think again. The flight from Melbourne takes off at 11.20 (11.20 AM). You will arrive in Chicago the same day at 19.45 (07.45 PM). Same day, but 24 hours later. That is all possible because you will cross the International Date Line.

The first leg of this monster journey is easy and requires no special anti jet lag preparations. Departure 11.20 (11.20 AM), arrival 16.35 (04.15 PM). Time difference between Melbourne and Auckland is two hours –it's two hours later in Auckland.

Second stretch: AKL to LAX, flight time 12 hours 45 minutes

Jet lag prevention:

For the second stretch of almost 13 hours, stop thinking about why it is getting night, while this day doesn't seem to end. Enjoy your reading, or the in-flight entertainment. Departure is at 18.35 (06.35 PM), arrival 11.20 (11.20 AM); hey that's the same time the plane took off from Melbourne yesterday. Or was it today? Is time going backwards?

The good part of this flight is that normal anti jet lag preparations are applicable. After take-off you will have some three hours to read, eat and for entertainment. Set your watch to LA time (not Chicago time). Convince your body that you will have a real long sleep and that when you wake up it will be around your regular waking up time, let's say 08.00.

Cabin lights will be switched on approximately 3 hours before expected landing time to give passengers plenty of time for breakfast. When you open the window shades enjoy the blue skies, the sunshine and the white clouds. It's morning!!

Third stretch LAX to ORD, flight time 4 hours
Jet lag prevention:

After such a long flight the aircraft needs a good inspection (and a good clean). That's why the stopover is more than an hour and a half. Use this time to get a quick shower and to stretch your legs. Walk around, don't sit down, be active.

Departure is 13.45 (01.45 PM), arrival 19.35 (07.35 PM). In winter it will be dark when you approach the airport. When you arrive in your hotel or at home it is time to go to bed. In mid summer it is still daytime on touch down, but even then you will not object to going to bed early.

The next day, resist temptations to be productive. Take it easy, make your business or other preparations and don't do anything drastic or important. And if you really *must* work, leave the office around lunchtime. Go home and take a nap.

The flight for a real no-jet lag pro is this one: a 30 hours trip from Singapore (SIN) to Ecuador (flying west through Amsterdam –long nights), spanning 13 time zones. Departure time on day 1 is 22.30 (10.30 PM). Flying time to Amsterdam is 12 hours. Arrival time in Amsterdam is therefore early in the morning at 06.00 on day 2. Here is the crunch; your flight to Quito does not leave Amsterdam until 22.30 (10.30 PM) that evening. Flying time to Quito with stops in Curacao (CUR) and Guayaquil (GUA) is 14.5 hours. Arrival time in Quito will be on the third day at 09.50 (09.50 AM).

This flight is a killer, unless you spend your time in Amsterdam to relax.

SIN-UIO: First stretch: SIN-AMS, flight time: 12 hours, 30 minutes
Jet lag prevention:
See the description of the Singapore-Jakarta leg of the previous flight. Enjoy dinner on board, prepare for the night, set your watch to Amsterdam time. Then convince your body to wake up early, sleep until 04.00 Amsterdam time. Have breakfast.

Stopover: 17 hours
That is a long stopover. What to do now?
The best thing to do is to extend your stopover in Amsterdam to a full day and night and to continue the journey the next day only.
However, if you *must* continue the same day, book a day room at the airport hotel inside the terminal building or in one of the hotels near the airport. Take it easy, do what you like, take a nap around 11.00. If in town, go for a walk. Have light meals during the day. Skip dinner and replace it with a light snack, because you will have dinner on board.

Second stretch: AMS-UIO, Flight time: 14 hours, 30 minutes
Jet lag prevention:
Be ready for a late dinner on board. If you have a window seat and if the sky is clear, you may want to enjoy the sight of the bright lights of Brighton,

Southampton and Portsmouth passing down below. After dinner, prepare for the night, set your watch to Quito time. Tell your body to wake up early because breakfast will be served before landing in Curacao (Amsterdam-Curacao is 9 hours). From Curacao you can have another nap.

In Quito, take a nap in the afternoon, then go to bed around 22.00 (10.00 PM). Between nap and bedtime you will love to walk in downtown Quito. Walk slowly, avoid running up and down stairs –or streets. The altitude (2,800 meters) will make your heart pound and your lungs will be short of oxygen. Your body will adjust to the altitude after three or four days.

The next flight plan, from Johannesburg (JNB) to Seattle (SEA) will keep you 'in the air', and a bit in several airports for a grueling 34 hours. The flight to the West Coast of the USA includes a stop in Lagos (LOS), Nigeria.

JNB to SEA: First stretch: JNB-LOS, flight time: 6 hours

Jet lag Prevention:
The time difference between Johannesburg and Lagos is one hour. Therefore, there is no need to make anti-jet lag preparations. Dinner will be served on this stretch. Enjoy!

Second stretch: LOS-JFK
Flight time: 11 hours 25 minutes
Jet lag prevention:
After stopping in Lagos for nearly two hours you will continue. Take off is scheduled at 00.45, arriving at JFK early in the morning a little after 6. Time difference between Lagos and New York is 6 hours. You may want to skip supper on board and 'retire' soon, taking full advantage of the long night flight.

If you can, break the journey in New York and continue to Seattle the next day. For those who are in a real hurry to get to Seattle, use the opportunity of the 11 hours stopover in JFK to take a shower. Try to find a quiet but light spot in the airport terminal to take in the morning atmosphere. Or store your luggage and go downtown to experience the Big Apple. Whatever you decide, take it easy.

Third stretch: JFK-SEA, flight time: 6 hours, 10 minutes
Jet lag prevention:
Departure from JFK is set at 17.15 (05.15 PM), arrival in Seattle's Tacoma International airport is 20.15 (08.15 PM). Time difference between NYC and SEA is four hours. By the time you arrive, simply go to bed, leaving the curtains open.

With the arrival of Super Jumbos (the Airbus 380 and the Boeing 787 Dreamliner) and other aircraft types capable of flying non-stop halfway around the globe, you may wonder how to combat jet lag in those situations.

The principle remains the same. For the 18 hours non-stop flight from Singapore to New York, for example you will apply the same procedure.
The flight leaves Changi Airport around noon. The arrival is scheduled at Newark at 17.00 (5.00 PM) the same day. The same day but 18 hours later! Don't worry about that detail; 18 hours is 18 hours and you will spend that time in broad daylight –if you fly during the northern hemisphere's summer season. The meal service will give you an indication of how much time you have between meals to be active and when to take naps; you will have three full meals. This is going to be a very lazy day. The economy class on this flight is an executive economy class with a nice seat and more space to move about. With this aircraft configuration you don't have to worry about someone in front of you reclining the seat. There is plenty of room between the

rows. Now you can open your laptop and do some work, stroll around the cabin and chat with passengers and crew. There is nothing to complain about the in-flight entertainment, so you will certainly not be bored. The trick on this journey is to stay on Singapore time until approximately halfway during the flight, after you have taken a refreshing afternoon nap. Leave the window shade open and be conscious of the afternoon atmosphere. You may even want to take several afternoon naps today, which is perfectly fine. What a luxury!

The return flight is just as interesting. It takes one hour longer to reach Singapore, flying across the North Pole. Take off is at 23.00 (11.00 PM) and arrival around 07.00 (07.00 AM) –two days later. Once again, don't worry about the two days later detail. The flight is only 19 hours while offering you the experience of the longest night in your life –probably. So, plan ahead, staying awake a little longer than usual. Go to bed after some three hours flying, scheduling a long sleep of six or seven hours.

When you wake up there will still be some nine hours to spend before arrival. Ignore all the clocks and convince yourself that it is still very early morning. Do some light chores, such as brushing your teeth or a bit of reading. Chances are that you will doze off again. Try to wake up around 04.00 or 05.00 AM Singapore time, ready to catch the first daylight and ready for a relaxing day in tropical Singapore.
It's good to take a little siesta (set the alarm and don't close the curtains) and in the evening, rather than enjoying Singapore's nightlife, to go to bed early.

Summary: It can be done!

Time Zones

F lying from north to south or south to north will see you cover no or only a few time zones. Even a very long flight such as from Santiago de Chile to New York (12 hours) will not cause jet lag. Passengers on this flight remain in the same time zone all the time during the USA winter season and in two time zones during the summer (because of Daylight Saving Time in the USA). Feeling exhausted and drowsy on arrival and weak in the knees is only the effect of the aircraft noise, the long sitting, the travel anxiety, and the lack of oxygen in the cabin.

Success in beating jet lag partly comes with knowing your current geographical location and knowing the time both in that location and at your destination. Without going into the theories of why things are the way they are on earth, flying east means that time passes faster so that the day seems shorter. Flying in the opposite direction (west) means that the day seems to last longer and that time passes slower.

The itinerary that your travel agent or the airline will give you together with your tickets may only contain the departure and arrival dates and times, but no information about the duration of the flight. Therefore you need more information. One source is the airline's in-flight magazine or its timetable. With a bit of luck you will be able to calculate the time at your destination, but very often you are an hour off, because of the applicable Daylight Saving Times. If in doubt a quick solution is to make a phone call, before your journey starts, to relatives, friends or business partners overseas:
"Hi, what time is it at your end? Woke you up? Oh, err, I had no idea, sorry!"

You could have asked your travel agent, but surprisingly, many travel agents have no clue about time zones and how to calculate time differences. Yet another option is to consult the flight tracking system, once you're airborne, usually projected between movies on board the aircraft. It gives the time at your current position, so that you know if it is happy hour or bedtime and also the time at your destination. The latter, as you know by now is the most important one to keep track of to avoid the misery of jet lag.

But if you want to know the exact time at your destination before setting off, you could download (for free) a simple piece of software, Earth Clock from 21stCenturypublishing or a similar software application (shareware) from Elanware (see the page with Internet links later on). The world maps from these companies are very nice and simple tools. The program from 21st-Centurypublishing allows you to point the cursor of your computer on any location on the globe and instantly you will see the time of day, compensated for Daylight Saving Times.

Basically, what happens when we travel in a jet, space shuttle, time capsule, what have you, is that time seems to go faster traveling east. It seems to be slower traveling west. Difficult to memorize? Try this one:

To east: short days, short nights
To west: long days, long nights

The explanation for this phenomenon has everything to do with the rotation of the earth. The world, as you may know, always rotates in an easterly direction. That's why the sun never rises in the west and never sets in the east. Very reliable. One could say that time come from the east, just like the Three Kings and several of our ancient cultures. An aircraft flying east is 'overtaking' the earth as it flies 'towards' time. That's why time going east seems to pass faster.
Similarly, an aircraft flying west is flying 'with the time'. That's why time going west seems to pass

slower. Apologies to academic circles for this unscientific explanation, but I hope it helps to explain something.

In the previous chapter we touched upon the International Date Line briefly. Understanding this imaginary line is very confusing for many human beings (including the author). To understand this phenomenon quickly you will need a globe or an atlas, or even better, the world clock software or something similar mentioned above.

To avoid that you have to get up from your seat, to switch on the computer or to get the atlas, we have put a photo on the cover of this book of good old and always beautiful mother Earth. If you have an atlas at home you will remember that on maps the globe is always shown with a grid of Latitudes and Longitudes (also called Meridians). The system with longitudes and latitudes was developed in the ancient times of wooden sailing ships to help captains, admirals and pirates navigate the globe when the Global Positioning System (GPS) was not even a dream for the future.

This classic system as we know it today was perfected in Britain when England not only ruled the waves but was about to expand into an empire. You will not be surprised to know therefore that the imaginary line (meridian) representing 0 degrees Longitude runs straight through Greenwich, a short distance east from London. That's where we find Greenwich Mean Time or GMT. A more modern notation is UTC, or Universal Time. World times are often referred to as so many hours + or – GMT or UTC.
Faraway from Greenwich, exactly on the opposite side of the Globe you will find the Longitude representing 180 degrees. That's where today changes into tomorrow or yesterday into today and that's how the identification 'International Date Line' was invented. West

from Greenwich the Longitudes are identified as so many degrees West. East from Greenwich they are known as so many degrees East.

On the cover photo of this book you will see the Globe without most of the grid. It's a bit of an unusual pose. We're looking from a spacecraft, if it were, hovering over the North Pole. The earth is slowly turning to the east, which is counter clockwise.

In the top part of the photo you can still see the outlines of Scandinavia, continental Europe, Russia, China and Asia. For your convenience we have highlighted the 0 degree Longitude meridian running across Britain and Greenwich.

Right from this meridian you can make out the snow and ice cover of Greenland. Going further you may recognize Canada, the US and a bit of Central America. In the lower part of the photo there is the vastness of the Pacific and the 180 degrees Longitude. It shows a zigzag pattern between Siberia and Alaska and also further south, not visible in the photo, where we find the Vanuatu islands and other Polynesian island groups.

Roughly every 20 degrees of Longitude constitutes a time zone. There are 24 time zones (because a day has 24 hours). In reality the time zones don't all run neat and straight along the meridians. That is because several countries, that geographically would fall in a certain time zone have opted to conform to a neighboring time zone. Singapore, for example does not follow Bangkok time but the time zone of Hong Kong and Manila.

Interestingly, Hong Kong time extends all the way to the west into the People's Republic of China. China has only one time zone, while logically it would need three.

Likewise, Spain and Portugal opted to follow West European Time, rather than Britain's time.

As we know from experience the date changes everywhere on earth at midnight, but at the International Dateline, the date changes all the time. Assuming that you are on a flight from Tokyo to Seattle (easterly direction), crossing the 180 degrees Longitude, let's say around 11.00 AM on a Saturday you will notice that suddenly it is yesterday again, Friday and also 11.00 AM.

Passengers of an aircraft, flying in a westerly direction at the same time and at the same spot will notice that for them today, which is Friday suddenly becomes tomorrow, Saturday.

Confused? That's fine as long as you're at home. When you travel be relaxed, be nice and marvel at the phenomenon.

Summary: No more talk, set your watch, it's time to take off!

Jet Lag Prevention Bullets

- Be relaxed: assume that everything can go wrong with your trip and at least some things definitely will
- Treat yourself to something nice
- Leave home at home
- Manage your time, be on time
- Dress casually
- Travel light
- Know the duration of your flight(s)
- Focus on the time at destination
- In flight sleep as long as you can or take as many cat naps as you can
- In flight cut back on coffee and alcohol
- Stay over if your entire journey will be more than 20 hours
- If you arrive in the morning, take a brief siesta (set the alarm!)
- Otherwise go to sleep at night
- Leave the curtains open

Jet lag prevention equipment:

- Eyeshades
- Earplugs or noise canceling headset
- Inflatable pillow

Related Websites

T he following websites provide information about jet lag in varying degrees of complexity and completeness:

www.bodyclock.com
www.flyana.com
www.jet lag.org
www.nojetlag.com
www.nomore-jet lag.com (the author's website)
www.Outsidein.co.uk

The World Clock software described in the previous chapters is available for free at:

www.21stcenturypublishing.com
www.elanware.com

Elanware's EarthWatch may also be downloaded from:

www.indonesia-ok.com. Look for the page Free Stuff

There are several air passenger associations representing the interests of us, air passengers. You may want to join one of those as a member. One of them is UK based IAPA (International Air Passenger Association):

www.iapa.com

A website that offers assistance with flight reservations, hotel bookings anywhere in the world and that has a host of travel planning tools is the Official Airline Guide, an authority in this field:

www.oag.com

After making your flight reservations, visit a site that offers information and learning about the safety record of airlines, quality of on-board service and the quality of food. There are ratings of airports around the world. All ratings are based on passenger experiences –you can submit your opinion too:

www.airlinequality.com

Rowing against the tide of the leading search engines is Copernic. You may consider downloading a free light version of Copernic, a very fast and complete search engine, with a multitude of search and filter options. It has enjoyed many positive reviews:

www.copernic.com

Printed in Great Britain
by Amazon.co.uk, Ltd.,
Marston Gate.